A Manual Of Instruction For Giving Swedish Movement And Massage Treatment

Hartvig Nissen

A MANUAL OF INSTRUCTION

FOR GIVING

SWEDISH MOVEMENT

AND

MASSAGE TREATMENT.

BY

PROF. HARTVIG NISSEN,

Director of the Swedish Health Institute, Washington, D. C.; Late Instructor
in Physical Culture and Gymnastics at the Johns Hopkins Uni-
versity, Baltimore, Md.; Author of "Health by
Exercise without Apparatus."

WITH 29 ORIGINAL WOOD ENGRAVINGS.

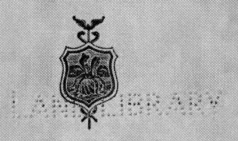

PHILADELPHIA AND LONDON:
F. A. DAVIS, PUBLISHER.
1889.

Philadelphia:
The Medical Bulletin Printing House,
1231 Filbert Street.

PREFACE.

SINCE my address on "Swedish Movement and Massage Treatment," delivered before the Clinical Society of Maryland in March, 1888, appeared in several medical journals, I have frequently been asked by the medical profession to write a manual, and also to give instructions on the subject.

Although there are numerous articles and books on massage, there are, to my knowledge, no manuals of Swedish movement and massage treatment in the English language which give any information how to apply the treatment in different diseases.

As such a treatise seems to be desirable, I have tried to write a practical hand-book, describing the most useful movements, many of these illustrated by cuts, and giving in addition prescriptions for their use in those cases where they are

(iii)

most likely to be successfully applied in the sick-room and without any apparatus.

I trust this will supply a need, and be accepted as a practical help in the treatment of the sick.

                                    HARTVIG NISSEN.

WASHINGTON, D.C.,
    May, 1889.

CONTENTS.

CHAPTER I.

CHAPTER II.

CHAPTER III.

(v)

CHAPTER IV.
DISEASES AND THEIR TREATMENT.
GROUP I.

CONTENTS.

THE SWEDISH MOVEMENT

AND

MASSAGE TREATMENT.

CHAPTER I.

HISTORY.

IT is a known fact that bodily exercise was used as a curative agent in the earliest days.

Æsculapius, Apollo's descendant, is said to have been the inventor of the art of gymnastics. Medea procured health and youth by gymnastics.

It was four hundred to five hundred years before Christ that Iccus, and later Herodicus, reduced bodily exercise to a system, and Herodicus made it a branch of medical science to preserve the health and cure diseases by the use of gymnastics, and among his many pupils was the famous Hippocrates.

Diocles, Praxagoras, Herophilus, Asclepiades, Athenæus, Celsus, and Galen recommended "movement treatment," and gave rules for it.

1 A

(1)

Mercurialis wrote in the sixteenth century a book, "De Arte Gymnastica," or the science of bodily exercise, which he divided into "Gymnastics for Athletes, for the Military, and for the Cure of Diseases," to which, as used by the Greeks and Romans, he gave especial attention, and pointed out the use of the different movements in different diseases, and also gave rules for their application in special cases.

Thomas Fuller, an English physician, published in 1704 "Medicina Gymnastica," treating of the power of exercise in preserving health and curing disease.

Clement J. Tissot, a French physician, who several times gained the prize of the Academie Royale de Chirurgie for his lectures, published in Paris, 1781, "Gymnastique Médicinale."

Gutsmuth, Jahn, Clias, and Spiess worked with energy to spread the German gymnastics or "Turnkunst," but paid no attention to gymnastics as used for the treatment of diseases.

As Herodicus observed the curative effects of gymnastics on his own delicate health, and thereby was brought to use movements in therapy, so did the Swede, Pehr Henrik Ling, in the beginning of this century, study the movement treatment because he had cured himself of rheumatism in the arm by gentle percussions.

Ling formerly had been only a fencing-master and instructor of gymnastics; but afterward, studying anatomy and physiology, and the influence of the movement and manipulations in different chronic diseases, he founded a system of gymnastics corresponding with the knowledge of physiology, which is universally known as "the Ling System," or the

"SWEDISH MOVEMENT TREATMENT."

By ardent study and labor, Ling succeeded at last in making his new ideas recognized, and in 1813 the first college for pedagogical, military, and medical gymnastics, called the "Royal Gymnastic Central Institute," was established in Stockholm at the expense and under the supervision of the Swedish Government, and Ling was its first President.

The principal studies for graduation at the present time are: Anatomy, Physiology, Pathology, Hygiene, Diagnosis, Principles of the Movement Treatment, and the use of exercises for general and local development.

Ling died in 1839. His pupils, Brandting,

Georgii, Liedback, and G. Indebetou, published Ling's theories, and by this means and through the many foreigners who studied at the Central Institute, of Stockholm, Ling's system soon became known in a great part of the world.

Dr. Joseph Schreiber, of Vienna (in his " Manual of Massage and Muscular Exercise," page 21), says: " The most powerful impetus, however, given to the revival of mechano-therapy originated with a Swede, the creator of the modern 'movement cure,' whose doctrines, spreading to England and to Germany, have, after many decades, and in spite of being marked by some extravagances, gained universal recognition."

De Ron, in St. Petersburg; Georgii, Indebetou, Bishop, and Roth, in London; Rothstein and Neumann, in Berlin; Richter, in Dresden; Schreber, in Leipzig; Melicher, in Vienna; Eulenburg, in Baden; Laisné, at the " Hôpital des Enfants Malads," in Paris; Taylor, in New York, and many others, established special institutions for movement treatment, and published their results partly in medical papers, partly in books.

CHAPTER II.

CLASSIFICATION OF MOVEMENTS.

ENDOWED with depth of thought as well as creative genius, fortified by sound scientific information, and sustained by an untiring devotion to his task, Ling was early led from result to result by a careful classification of movements and by a scientific examination of their different results. Ling distinguished, in the first instance, between

"ACTIVE" AND "PASSIVE" MOVEMENTS,

active movements being such as the subject performs entirely by voluntary muscular contraction, and *passive movements* such as the subject takes no part in beyond allowing the operator to *move* the whole or any portion of his body—as *flexion*, *extension*, and *rotation*—and to manipulate it, as in *stroking*, *kneading*, *pressing*, *percussing*, etc.

These simple movements Ling combined into

RESISTIVE, OR DUPLEX MOVEMENTS,

viz., *active-passive*, or "concentric duplex" movements, such as the patient makes, while the

(5)

operator resists, and *passive-active*, or "eccentric duplex" movements, such as the operator overcomes, while the patient resists; duplex, because two individuals engage in it; concentric, because the patient's muscles have to overcome a resistance which prevents flexion—a movement toward the trunk; eccentric, because the force acts in a direction away from the body.

The word *massage* means *kneading*, but is now generally used to describe the *handling* and *manipulating* of the flesh, as in *stroking, pressing, kneading, percussing,* etc.

Thus "massage" is only a part of the "*passive*" *movements*, and constitutes a very small part of the "Swedish movement treatment."

The Purpose of this Manual.

It would be impossible for any one to gain a thorough knowledge of this system, and how, understandingly, to give a full treatment, from a brief manual like the present one.

Two or three years of hard study is required at the Royal Central Institute of Stockholm in order to be graduated there.

But there are hundreds of cases where the *passive movements*, together with a few of the most useful *resistive movements*, will not only give a great relief, but even effect a cure, when applied judiciously and according to physiological laws.

For the treatment of those cases where the doctor himself, or an operator under the doctor's direction, will apply the " movements," or what is commonly called the " massage," in the sickroom, and without the use of apparatus, it is the object of this manual to describe.

There is also another reason why a manual of this kind is necessary, namely, a great many physicians, as well as others, consider this treatment to be a humbug, but this is due partly to prejudice and partly to their entire ignorance of the system.

Others think that "Swedish movements" mean regular active gymnastics, and think of " massage" only as a kind of "magnetism or rubbing."

Again, some physicians, anxious to find out what there is in this treatment, have employed persons calling themselves "masseurs" to apply massage to patients. As a natural result of this, in many cases the treatment proved of no value whatever, and in some instances actual harm was done.

It has happened more than once to the author
of this book that he has been called in by physicians to apply " massage " to patients who were
already suffering with a high fever, and he inva-
riably declined to do so. In one of these cases
the patient died the following day. Had the
physician's request been acceded to, the massage
treatment would have been accredited with has-
tening or causing the sick man's death.

At other times the writer has asked the physician in charge what the illness was, and has
been told that it was unnecessary for him to
know.

*Some physicians seem to have the idea that we
specialists are their rivals and their opponents.
Still, we have frequently repeated that we are
not physicians and do not practice medicine.*

*We are specialists, and, as such, necessarily
physiologists, and have the practical experience
gained by the practice of many years in this one
branch.*

*But it is co-operation between the medical pro-
fession and the specialists which is desirable and
necessary in order to produce the best results.*

Therefore, it is the aim of this little book to
enlighten those who want to know, and to show

how the treatment should be applied in different cases.

Swedish movements and massage are based on plain physiological laws, and have nothing in common with "magnetism," nor is it "regular gymnastics," nor "rubbing."

When the physician desires to have this treatment applied to a patient, and does not want to execute it himself, he should always take care that the one employed thoroughly understands his business.

As Dr. D. Graham says: "It is not to be wondered at that many a shrewd, superannuated auntie, and others who are out of a job, having learned the meaning of the word massage, immediately have it printed on their cards, and continue their 'rubbin,' just as they have always done."

Finally, it must be said that it is not our claim to cure all kinds of diseases by movements. Far from that. Some diseases, it is true, can be cured quicker by this method than by any other. In most cases, however, it has to be used together with medical treatment, for the same reason that electricity, baths, etc., are very often employed to bring about a cure. In other cases it should be

resorted to only as an after-cure, or as a means
of exercise.

WHO SHOULD APPLY THE TREATMENT.

After a little study and practice no physician
should have any trouble in treating a case of
neurasthenia, insomnia, acute muscular rheumatism, sprains, etc., but he will hardly have either
the facilities, dexterity, patience, or time to treat
sciatica, ankylosis of years' standing, confirmed
constipation, heart disease, or spinal curvatures,
etc.   A specialist should always be called for the
treatment of such cases, for he will not be dis-
couraged by the apparent lack of success in the
beginning (often extending over months), and
has, besides, apparatus by the use of which he
can facilitate the cure; or may, indeed, have an
establishment of his own wherein trained assistants devote all their time and energies to this
method alone.

THE VARIETY OF MOVEMENTS AND DURATION

of treatment is of great importance.

It is an utterly false idea that "massage" is
merely "rubbing," and needs only to be applied
by a strong hand and for an hour's time.

As Dr. D. Graham says: " The argument, too often used, that massage can do no harm, if it does no good, is a dangerous one.   When a man understands one branch of the medical profession well, one of the commonest errors is to suppose that he understands all the rest equally as well, as if our knowledge of massage, like everything else, did not come through experience."

For instance, in a case of synovitis, or glandular enlargement, the manipulations should always be directed *centripetally*, toward the heart; but in case of insomnia, or very *painful neuralgia*, the manipulations should be directed downward, from the shoulder toward the fingers, from the hips toward the toes, in order to ease and quiet the nerves.   In cases of *congestion*, movements must be applied to drive the blood from the part; in other cases, as *anæmia*, it is necessary to increase the flow of blood to the part.

Now, for instance, there are two patients, a delicate woman and a strong, robust man, both suffering with rheumatism.   It might be fair to treat the man for about an hour, but it would surely be too much to let the woman undergo the same treatment for the same length of time.

Always bear in mind that the old maxim, "If a little does good, more will do more good," is an exploded theory. A good operator can accomplish more in fifteen minutes than a poor one in an hour.

How Often the Treatment Should be Repeated.

It is a mistake, frequently made by physicians, to recommend their patients to try movement or massage treatment only two or three times a week, "because they cannot stand it," or, "they are too weak to try it oftener."

The weaker a patient is the oftener he ought to have the treatment. The treatment should be applied at least once a day, and sometimes twice, in order to derive the most benefit from it. The effect which is derived from one treatment should not be lost before the next treatment is applied.

It is the treatment which builds up the patient's strength, but if only tried once in a while he will feel tired and stiff a day or two afterward, and naturally conclude that the treatment does him harm—just as a man who takes a ten-mile horseback ride once a week feels sore and stiff each time, and never gets over it until he repeats the riding several times weekly.

To a weak patient the treatment has to be given very gently in the beginning, and, providing it is applied regularly, may soon be increased in force, and thus more vigor is given to the patient.

How to be Dressed

when under treatment is a frequent question. In all cases where the manipulations are to be directed *centripetally*, it is necessary to strip the body; but in other cases it is preferred that it should be clothed, as that will lessen the pain which sometimes is produced by the manipulations, and the skin (not being the seat of the trouble) will be more protected.

The dress should be as light as possible, and all tight clothing dispensed with.

Physiological Effects of Movements.

These may be divided into two groups:—

First. Purely mechanical effects to secure the removal of lymph, exudations, extravasations, etc., softening of exudations, and loosening of adhesions.

Second. Increased circulation by stimulating the muscular and nervous system, causing mole-

cular changes, changes in sensation, and changes
in the nutritive functions.

Dr. J. Schreiber says: "We understand by

PASSIVE MOVEMENTS

all movements performed by the physician upon
the patient, the latter remaining passive.

"The following results are obtained:—

"1. Extravasations occurring about dislocated
joints are, by pressing and rubbing the tendons
and ligaments in which they are imbedded,
finally liquefied, and thus more quickly absorbed.

"2. In stiffness of joints the contracted muscles
and tendons are forcibly but gradually elongated,
and any existing exudations or vegetations within
the joints are disintegrated and absorbed.

"3. By the forcible stretching of the muscles
their nerves are likewise stretched, molecular
changes being thus set up in both.

"4. Forced extension of the muscles causes
pressure on their blood and lymphatic vessels,
thus accelerating the circulation.

"5. Finally, such muscles as have by rheumatic
or neuralgic pains been kept in a state of inac-
tivity have some of their much-needed exercise
restored to them. Passive movements thus form

in certain diseases, as in neuralgia and rheumatism, the introduction, as it were, for the more painful active motions which have to follow."

Dr. D. Graham, "Treatise on Massage," page 23, says: "In 1844 the Supreme Medical Board of Russia appointed two members of the Medical Council to inquire into the merits of the movement and manipulation treatment as practiced by M. de Ron, one of Ling's disciples at St. Petersburg, who had been using it then for a period of twelve years. From the highly commendatory report of the Councillors we quote the following: 'All passive movements, or those which are executed by an external agent upon the patient, as well as active ones produced by the effort of the voluntary muscles, and the different positions with the aid of apparatus or without it, are practiced according to a strictly defined method, and conducted rationally, since they are based upon mechanical as well as anatomical principles.'

"*Experience teaches us the usefulness of the institution, as many patients thus treated have recovered their health after having suffered from diseases which could not be cured by other remedies.*"

THE ACTIVE AND RESISTIVE MOVEMENTS

cause an increased flow of blood to the muscles and soft parts, increasing thereby the circulation and removing accumulation of tissue waste. They cause resorption of exudations, transudations, and infiltrations, and a separation of adhesions in tendon-sheaths and in joints. They increase the oxidizing powers of the blood; they relieve the congestion of the brain, lungs, intestines, uterus, liver, and kidneys, by increasing the flow of blood to the muscles; they stimulate directly the sympathetic nervous system, thus increasing secretion, and reflexly the activity of unstriped muscle-fibres, and so relieve various functional derangements.

And they educate morbidly affected muscles to convert abnormal into normal actions and to suppress useless movements.

Thus movement treatment influences the living organism—

First, by increasing the circulation, respiration, and temperature, improving the digestion, absorption, and nutrition, and facilitating excretion.

Second, the muscles become developed, the bones and the whole human frame better proportioned.

Third, appetite is increased, and food is taken with greater relish.

Fourth, sleep is facilitated.

Fifth, the brain acts more vigorously and is freed from psychical depression.

Sixth, relieves pain and removes congestion.

The Movements May be Spoken of as

"Strengthening" movements, such as flexion, extension, torsion, etc.

"Stimulating" movements, as percussion, vibration, etc.

"Quieting" movements, as rotation, friction, etc.

"Derivative" movements, with special movements of the extremities.

"Purgative" movements, as kneading, pressing, and active movements of the abdominal muscles.

Some movements have a special effect on the "respiration," others on the "circulation," etc.

CHAPTER III.

POSITIONS.

Ling distinguished between five different fundamental positions, viz. :—

Standing.
Kneeling.
Sitting.
Lying.
Hanging.

These he subdivided into a number of starting positions with the arms, legs, trunk, and head, as

Standing—*hands on hips,*
arms horizontal,
arms vertical,
Sitting—*astride sitting,*
forward bent sitting,
Lying—*reclining,*
knees bent,
on back lying,
on front lying,

which, combined in various ways, make nearly

(19)

. twelve thousand positions in which the different movements may be either taken or given. And so the number of movements may be said to be endless, to suit each particular ailment.

MOVEMENTS OF THE ARMS.

A. *Passive Movements.*

1. *Centripetal stroking, pressing, kneading, circular friction,* and *vibratory friction* are all to be given from the tip of the fingers toward the shoulder.

Grasp the patient's finger with your thumb and two first fingers, and make a firm pressing and stroking movement upward toward the hand; at the same time let your fingers glide in a circular way round the patient's finger, describing the motions of a screw. Let your fingers glide easily back to the starting-point (the tip of the patient's finger), and repeat the motions fifteen to twenty times on each finger.

In treating the hand, use your fingers and the palm in pressing and stroking, and continue the same way toward the elbow. Then knead the muscles from the fingers toward the elbow by picking up each group of muscles with the one hand (Fig. 1, A), and when releasing the grasp

make an upward pressure with the other hand
(Fig. 1, B, *kneading*).

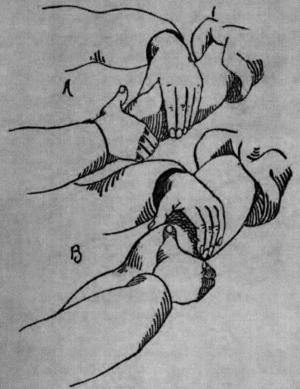

FIG. 1.—KNEADING.

Again, grasp the hand with both of yours, and
make upward pushing movements, constantly

moving the hands and fingers in a circular direction, thereby making a sideways friction together
with the upward stroke (*circular friction*, Fig. 2).

Now, let the patient's arm rest in your left
hand, and with your right make a pressure and
shaking movement of the different muscles, constantly gliding upward (*vibratory friction*). The

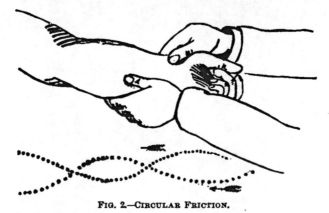

FIG. 2.—CIRCULAR FRICTION.

same movements are to be made from the elbow
to the shoulder.

When the whole arm has been worked over in
this manner from *four* to *ten* times, make firm
strokes from the fingers to the shoulder, clasping
the limb around with both your hands, from *five*
to *ten* times.

These movements are given in order to remove lymph, exudations, transudations, etc., and to effect the solution and removal of adhesions.

2. *Nerve Compression.*—Grasping the limb with both hands, a firm pressure is made around and down the whole arm, from the shoulder to the fingers. Repeated three to five times (Fig. 3).

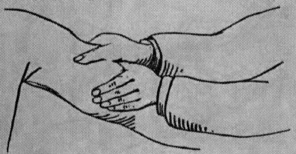

FIG. 3.—NERVE COMPRESSION.

This stimulates the nerves and increases the circulation of the blood.

3. *Muscle Rolling.*—Grasping the limb with the palms of both hands (Fig. 4), and making a quick, alternate pushing-and-pulling motion, and gradually gliding downward from the shoulder, the muscles of the arm will be rolled against each other, whereby the circulation of the blood is very much increased. Repeated three to five times.

4. *Slapping.*—This is performed with the palm of both hands, with a light motion of the wrist-joint, and the whole arm is slapped from the shoulder downward from three to five times. Useful in rheumatism, lameness, cold hands, etc.

5. *Friction* is performed with the fingers and palm of the hand from the shoulder and down-

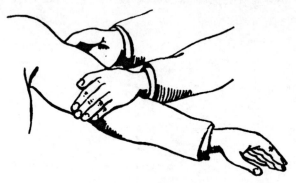

FIG. 4.—MUSCLE ROLLING.

ward, grasping around the limb with both hands, repeated ten to thirty times. This should be done in slow time. This has a quieting effect on the nerves, and by irritating the walls of the blood-vessels the circulation of the blood in the capillaries is stimulated.

Nerve compression, muscle rolling, slapping, and *friction* are frequently used together as an excellent way to increase the circulation of the blood and quiet the nerves.

6. *Percussion* is performed with the edge of the extended fingers (Fig. 5), which are kept loose, and with a quick motion of the wrist-joint the fingers are flung *across* the muscles from the shoulder toward the hand.

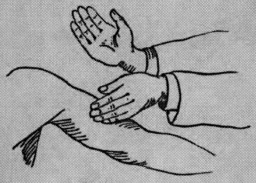

FIG. 5.—PERCUSSION.

7. *Beating* is performed with the clenched fist (Fig. 6, A) on and around the fleshy part of the limb with a loose and light movement of the wrist-joint (Fig. 6, B).

These two motions have a stimulating effect, and are useful in lameness and weakness of the muscles, in rheumatism, etc.

8. *Vibration.*—The operator takes hold of the

patient's hand and makes a slight pull and a very rapid vibration (shaking) of the whole arm. Repeated three to five times. This has a stimu-

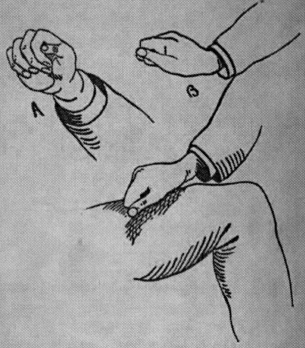

FIG 6.—BEATING.

lating and strengthening effect on the nerves and also on the respiration.

9. *Finger Rotation.*—The joint between the

finger and hand is fixed by the operator's one hand, and with his other the finger is rotated in its joint, first ten to twenty times one way, then as many times the other way.

10. *Hand rotation* is performed by taking hold of the wrist with one hand and of the fingers with the other hand, and describing a circle in the wrist-joint from ten to twenty times each way.

11. *Forearm Rotation.*—The patient's elbow is fixed in the operator's one hand, who, with the other hand, takes hold of the patient's wrist (see Fig. 9) and moves the forearm, which is kept on a right angle, in a circle in the elbow-joint, from ten to twenty times each way.

These movements are used in stiffness of the joints and cold hands, and as derivative from the chest and head.

12. For the same purpose is given *arm*, *hand*, and *finger* flexion, "passive," by alternately bending and stretching the joints.

13. *Arm Rotation* (A, *Single*).—The operator takes hold of the patient's shoulder with one hand and of his elbow with the other hand, moves the arm forward, upward, backward, and down and reverse, so as to describe a circle of

the shoulder-joint, from five to ten times each way.

This increases the circulation and limbers the shoulder-joint, and has a derivative effect on the chest and head.

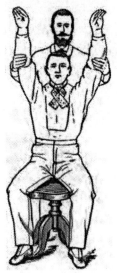

FIG. 7.—FORWARD ARM ROTATION.

14. *Forward Arm Rotation — Sitting* (B, *Double*).—The operator, standing behind the patient, the latter resting his back against the operator's chest, then takes hold of his arms just below the elbows and moves them in a

circle forward, upward, sideways, and down, from ten to twenty times (Fig. 7).

This expands the chest and has a great effect on the respiration and the circulation.

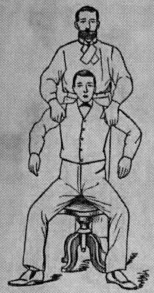

FIG. 8.—SHOULDER ROTATION AND CHEST LIFTING.

15. *Shoulder Rotation and Chest Lifting—Sitting.*—The patient sits on a stool or box, and the operator, standing behind, takes hold under and in the front of the patient's shoulders, moves them upward, backward, and down, at the same

time pressing his chest against the patient's back. Repeated eight to fourteen times (Fig. 8).

This is a mild but effective movement in weakness of the lungs and heart, as it deepens the inspiration followed by a stronger expiration,

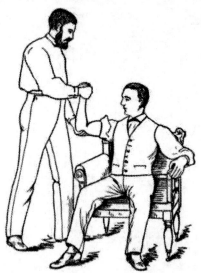

FIG. 9.—ARM FLEXION AND EXTENSION.

thereby stimulating the flow of venous blood to the heart.

B. *Resistive Movements.*

16. *Hand and Finger Flexion and Extension.* —Position as in rotations. Resistance is made

alternately by the operator and the patient. This develops and strengthens the muscles of the fore-arm, hand, and fingers, and increases the flow of blood to them.

17. *Arm Flexion and Extension.* — Position as in "forearm" rotation. The patient first stretches and bends his arm, in the elbow-joint, during the resistance of the operator, "active-passive." Then the operator stretches and bends the arm, during the resistance of the patient, "passive-active." Repeated from three to ten times (Fig. 9).

This develops and strengthens the flexor and extensor muscles of the arm and increases the circulation.

18. *Vertical Arm Flexion and Extension—Sitting.*—The operator stands behind and a little higher than the patient and takes hold of both his hands, resisting the patient when he bends and stretches his arms, "active-passive," in a slow movement, the elbows being kept well out to the side. The operator's knee should be pressed against the patient's back with a small pillow between. Repeated from five to fourteen times (Fig. 10).

This strengthens the muscles of the chest and

back as well as of the arms, and it expands and deepens the chest.

19. *Horizontal Arm Flexion and Extension—Sitting.*—The patient's arms are raised horizon-

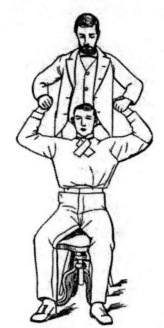

FIG. 10.—VERTICAL ARM FLEXION AND EXTENSION.

tally and kept well back, with the forearms sharply bent upon them; the operator, standing behind, pressing his chest against the patient's back, takes hold of both his wrists (Fig. 11) and resists, when the patient stretches and bends his arms at the elbow-joints, "active-passive." Repeated from five to ten times.

This strengthens the muscles of the upper

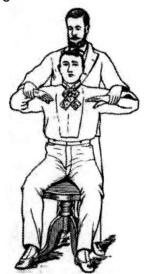

FIG. 11.—HORIZONTAL ARM FLEXION AND EXTENSION.

arms; it expands the chest and is a good respiratory and derivative movement.

20. *Horizontal Arm Separation and Closing—Sitting.*—The operator, standing in front of the patient, who holds his arms straight out to the

2*

sides, takes hold of his wrists and pulls the arms forward under resistance by the patient, "passive-active." Then the patient brings his arms back to the former position resisted by the operator, "active-passive." Repeated from five to ten times (Fig. 12).

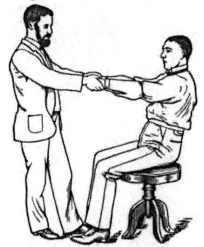

FIG. 12.—HORIZONTAL ARM SEPARATION AND CLOSING.

This acts on the muscles of the back of the shoulders, whereby the shoulders are straightened; it has a good effect on the respiration and the circulation.

21. *Lateral Arm Elevation and Depression.*—The operator, standing behind the patient, takes

hold of his forearms, which are hanging down,
and resists when the patient raises his arms sideways, upward, and when he brings them down
again, "active-passive." The elbows should be
kept straight. Repeated from five to ten times
(Fig. 13).

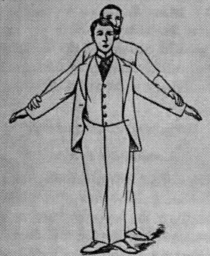

FIG. 13.—LATERAL ARM ELEVATION AND DEPRESSION.

This is a very effective movement to widen the
chest and to strengthen the muscles of the
shoulders and upper arms. It has a good effect
on the respiration and circulation.

22. *Arm Torsion.*—The patient takes hold of

the middle of a stick with one hand and keeps his arm straight. The operator takes hold of each end of the stick and resists the patient when he *twists* his arm outward and inward, "active-passive." This movement may be changed by letting the patient resist when the operator twists the arm, "passive-active." Repeated from five to ten times.

This is used in stiffness of the shoulder-joint and in abnormal enervations of the muscles of the arm, and is a good derivative from the chest and head.

MOVEMENTS OF THE LEGS.

A. *Passive Movements.*

23. *Centripetal stroking, pressing, kneading, circular friction,* and *vibratory friction* should all be applied in the same manner as to the arms, beginning with the toes and gradually proceeding toward the hip. (See Figs. 1 and 2.)

24. *Nerve compression, muscle rolling, slapping,* and *friction* from the hip toward the foot are similar to those movements given the arms, as above described. (See Figs. 3 and 4.)

25. *Percussion,* as applied to the arms. (See Fig. 5.)

26. *Beating*, as applied to the arms. (See Fig. 6.)

27. *Vibration.*—The operator, taking hold of the patient's heel and ankle, makes a slight pulling and shaking movement of the whole limb.

This has a stimulating effect on the nerves.

28. *Foot Rotation* (A, *Single*).—The operator

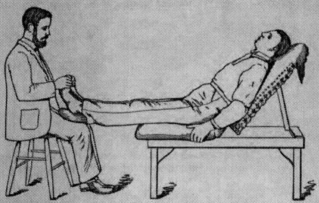

FIG. 14.—FOOT ROTATION, DOUBLE.

fixes the patient's ankle with one hand, and, taking hold of the toes with the other hand, moves the foot around in a circle ten to twenty times one way, and reverses.

This is useful in stiffness of the ankle-joint and cold feet.

29. B, *Double.*—The patient, in a lying or

reclining position, rests the back of his heels against a cushion. The operator, sitting in front of the patient, takes hold of his toes (Fig. 14) and moves both feet in a quick circle twenty to thirty times the one way, and reverse. The legs should be kept straight during the motion.

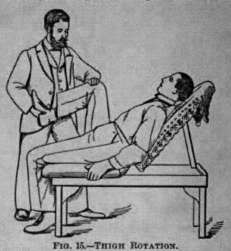

FIG. 15.—THIGH ROTATION.

This has a very good effect on the circulation, and, by increasing the flow of blood to the feet, acts as a good derivative from other organs.

30. *Foot and toe flexion, passive,* is generally used in connection with the rotation.

31. *Thigh Rotation.*—The operator takes hold

of the patient's foot with one hand and of his bent knee with the other hand (Fig. 15); the knee is now pressed upward, then moved outward and downward so as to describe a circle in the hip-joint; the knee should not be moved to pass the middle line of the body Should be repeated from five to ten times each way.

This is very useful in equalizing the circulation and as a derivative from diseases in the pelvis and abdomen, as well as to limber the hip-joint.

B. *Resistive Movements.*

32. *Foot Flexion and Extension* (A, *Single*, and B, *Double*, Fig. 14).—Positions as in *foot rotation.* The patient bends and stretches his feet during resistance by the operator, "active-passive."

These strengthen the muscles of the calf and foot and limber the ankle-joint. It is a good derivative movement, and is especially beneficial in cases of cold feet.

33. *Leg Flexion and Extension.*—The operator, standing by the side of the patient, takes hold of his heel with one hand and of the ball of the foot with the other hand (Fig. 16). The leg is bent without resistance, and then the

patient stretches it out, when the operator resists
by pressing the leg upward and slightly giving
way till it is perfectly straight, "active-passive."
Repeated from five to ten times.

This is an excellent movement to strengthen
the extensor muscles of the whole limb, and also

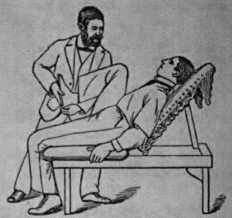

FIG. 16.—LEG FLEXION AND EXTENSION.

as a derivative from diseases of the pelvis and
abdomen.

34. *Upward Knee Traction.*—The operator
takes hold of the back of the patient's heel with
one hand and on the front of his foot with the
other hand and resists, when the patient bends
his leg—pulling his knee upward—by holding

it straight, and slightly giving way till it is doubled up; it is again straightened without resistance. Repeated five to ten times (Fig. 17).

This movement strengthens the flexor muscles of the leg and the muscles of the abdomen, and thus has a purgative effect.

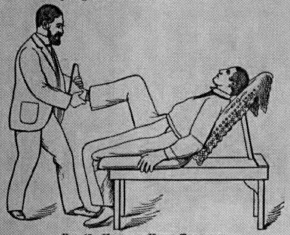

FIG. 17.—UPWARD KNEE TRACTION.

35. *Knee Flexion and Extension.*—The operator, sitting by the side of the patient, whose thigh is resting on the operator's knee (Fig. 18), fixes the patient's knee with one hand and takes hold with the other hand around his ankle, resisting, when the patient bends, and stretches his knee. Repeated five to ten times.

B³

This is useful in stiffness and weakness of the knee-joint and to strengthen the muscles of the thigh. It has a derivative effect.

36. *Leg Elevation and Depression—Lying.*— The patient, keeping his knee straight, raises his leg upward by bending the hip-joint, the operator making slight resistance with his hands on

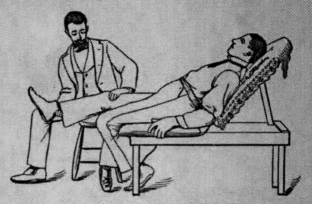

FIG. 18.—KNEE FLEXION AND EXTENSION.

the patient's knee, "active-passive." Then the patient resists, while the operator presses the limb down again, "passive-active" (Fig. 19). Repeated five to ten times.

This may also be performed with both legs at the same time when the patient is young and strong.

The muscles of the abdomen, the flexor muscles of the thigh, and the extensor muscles of the leg are hereby brought into play. It has a purgative as well as a derivative effect.

37. *Leg Separation and Closing—Lying.*— The operator takes hold of the patient's ankle

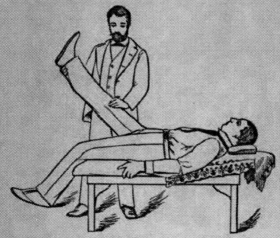

FIG. 19.—LEG ELEVATION AND DEPRESSION.

and resists him when he brings his leg out to the side, "active-passive." Then the patient resists while the operator presses the leg into its former position, "passive-active." Repeated four to eight times.

This strengthens the muscles of the hip and

thigh and is a good derivative from the organs of the pelvis.

38. *Bent Knee Separation and Closing.*—The patient bends his knees to a sharp angle, the feet resting on the bed or chair; the operator puts his hands on the outside of each knee (Fig. 20) and

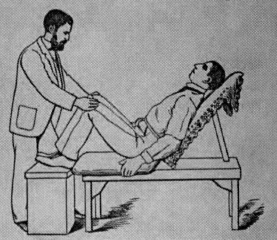

FIG. 20.—BENT KNEE SEPARATION AND CLOSING.

resists when the patient separates the knees. Then the operator changes his hands to the inside of the knees and resists while the patient closes them, "active-passive." Repeated three to five times.

Now the movement is reversed so that the

operator separates and closes the knees when the patient resists, "passive-active." Repeated three to five times.

The feet should be kept firm in their place during the moving of the knees.

This brings into play the muscles of the hips, pelvis, and thighs, and is a derivative movement.

39. *Leg Torsion.*—The patient keeps his legs straight and the operator takes hold of the feet and resists while the patient twists his legs out and inward by separating and closing the feet, the heels being kept together. Repeated five to ten times.

This is useful in stiffness and weakness of the hip-joint and as a derivative from the organs of the pelvis.

MOVEMENTS OF THE TRUNK.

A. *Passive Movement.*

40. *Chest Kneading and Friction.*—First make a few strokes with both hands from the middle of the chest—the sternum—and out to the side. Then knead and vibrate the skin and the muscles all over the chest, always commencing at the middle and working outward, and finish with frictions.

41. *Chest Slapping.*—The operator, standing

in front of the patient, brings his hands on the back of the patient's shoulders and slaps him over the traction of the lungs, then moving forward under the arms to the chest and all over the chest up to the shoulders. Repeated three to six times.

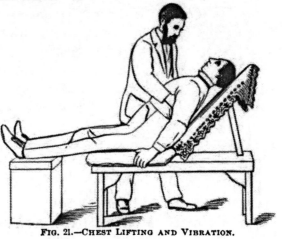

FIG. 21.—CHEST LIFTING AND VIBRATION.

This is useful in weakness and emphysema of the lungs, organic diseases of the heart, and in nervous palpitation.

42. *Chest Lifting and Vibration.*—The operator, standing in front of the patient, puts his hands on each side and under the shoulders of the patient, then lifts him slightly (Fig. 21) and,

by shaking his hands, effects a vibration of the whole trunk. Repeated four to eight times at short intervals.

This stimulates the lungs and heart.

43. *Stomach friction* is made with both hands all over the abdomen from the middle and out to

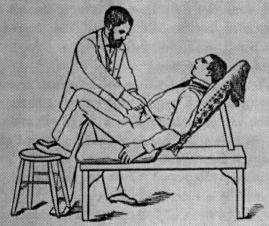

FIG. 22.—STOMACH KNEADING.

the sides several times, followed with an upward stroke with the one hand on the right side and over to the left in the direction of the ascending and transverse colon, and then a downward stroke with the other hand on the left side in the direction of the descending colon. Repeated four to eight times.

Useful in indigestion, dyspepsia, constipation.

44. *Stomach Kneading.*—With the slightly bent knuckles of the fingers an alternate pressure is made with both hands all over the abdomen several times (Fig. 22). Then a kneading and rolling of the flesh and muscles is made in a circle from the right upward, over to the left and downward, in the direction of the ascending, transverse, and descending colon. Especially useful in constipation.

45. *Stomach Vibrations.*—The operator presses his slightly bent fingers under the patient's ribs on the left side and applies a rapid vibration on the ventricle; the hands should be moved so as to apply the vibration all over the left hypo-chondriac. Repeated three to six times, and followed by a stomach friction.

Useful in cases of dyspepsia and chronic catarrh of the stomach.

46. *Bowel Vibration—Standing.*—The operator, standing behind the patient, puts both his hands on the patient's abdomen, and by a rapid pushing and pulling motion of his hands an effective vibration is applied to the whole bowel. Repeated three to six times.

Very useful in constipation.

47. *Bowel Concussion—Lying.* — The operator's both hands are placed on the patient's bowel, and a pressure is made. Then the hands are quickly taken off, allowing the abdomen to spring back like a rubber ball. Repeated three to five times.

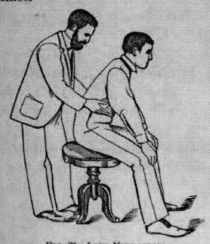

FIG. 23.—LOIN VIBRATION.

This strengthens the abdominal muscles and the digestive power.

48. *Loin Vibration—Sitting.*—The operator, standing behind the patient, who sits on a lounge or box, presses his hands on each side of the patient just above his hips (Fig. 23), and

3c

applies a very rapid alternate pushing and pulling movement with his hands (reciprocating
vibration). The hands must be firm and not
glide on the flesh. Repeated three to six times
at short intervals.

This has a very stimulating effect on the
liver and stomach and on the lungs and the
diaphragm.

49. *Loin Traction—Lying.* — The operator
presses his hands on each side and under the
loin of the patient, and pulls his hands forcibly
forward, just above the hips. Repeated four to
ten times.

Useful in cases of indigestion and constipation.

50. *Breech beating* is applied with the
clenched fist of the one hand from the small
of the back, down the sacral bone, and all over
the buttocks to the beginning of the thigh, in
slow time. Repeated five to eight times.

This acts on the sacral nerves and is useful in
weakness of the bladder and sexual organs and
in constipation.

51. *Back kneading, vibration, and friction* is
applied from the base of the skull downward,
and from the spinal column outward to the sides,
all over the back (Fig. 24). A very good

movement in connection with these is to put the
heel of the hands on the spinal column at the
neck and apply a rapid shaking movement,
letting the one hand slowly glide downward to
the end of the spine.   The whole manipulation

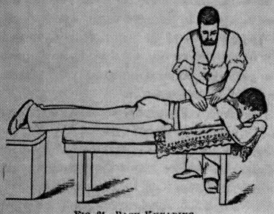

FIG. 21.—BACK KNEADING.

should always be followed by long and slow
frictions on both sides of the spinal column.

These movements increase the circulation,
stimulate the action of the nerves, and have a
very soothing and quieting effect.

52. *Spinal Nerve Compression.*—The operator
presses with his fingers first on the one side of
the spinal column and then on the other side

from the neck and downward. Repeated three to six times.

Relieves backache and stimulates the nerve centres.

53. *Back percussion* is applied with the edge of both hands alternately from the neck and downward on both sides of the spinal column. On the upper part of the back, from the shoulders to the lower end of the lungs, the percussion may also be applied outward to the sides. Repeated six to ten times.

This has a very stimulating and strengthening effect on the nerve-centre.

54. *Trunk Rotation—Astride Sitting.*—The patient sits astride over a box or lounge, while the operator, standing behind, takes hold of the patient's shoulders and moves his trunk from the waist, describing as large a circle as possible, first to the left, then to the right, the patient being perfectly passive. Repeated eight to sixteen times each way.

This has a good effect on the spine and the portal system, and is a quieting movement.

B. *Resistive Movements.*

55. *Trunk Torsion—Sitting.*—The patient sits on a stool, or lounge, with hands on hips. The

operator, standing behind, puts his right hand on the front of the patient's right shoulder and his left hand on the back of his left shoulder, and resists the patient when he turns or twists his trunk to the left. (See Fig. 25.) Then the

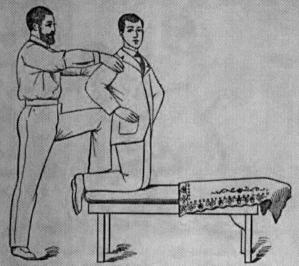

FIG. 25.—TRUNK TORSION—KNEELING.

operator changes his grip, reverses the hands, and resists when the patient turns to the right. Repeated four to eight times to each side.

56. *Trunk Torsion—Kneeling.*—The patient kneels on a lounge or bed with hands on hips.

The operator, standing behind and fixing the patient's back with his one knee, takes hold and resists, as in the former movement. Repeated four to eight times (Fig. 25).

Both of these movements have a good effect on the spine, the nerves, and circulation; the

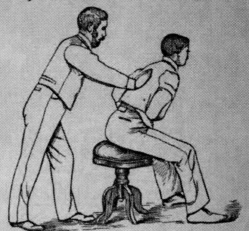

FIG. 26.—FORWARD TRUNK FLEXION AND EXTENSION.

former has a special effect on the respiration and the latter on the digestion, by strengthening and elevating the muscles of the abdomen.

57. *Forward Trunk Flexion and Extension—Sitting.*—The patient, sitting on a lounge or box, with hands on hips, bends forward, and, while

rising up to the former position, the operator puts his hands on the patient's back and resists him (Fig. 26). Repeated four to eight times.

This strengthens the muscles of the back and straightens the spine.

C. *Active Movements.*

58. *Trunk Elevation—Lying.*—The patient, lying on a lounge or bed, with the lower legs

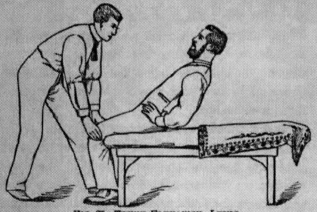

FIG. 27.—TRUNK ELEVATION—LYING.

hanging down, raises his body to a sitting position, the operator fixing the patient's knees (Fig. 27). Repeated two to six times.

This strengthens the abdominal muscles and is a purgative movement.

MOVEMENTS OF THE HEAD.

A. *Passive Movements.*

59. *Head Percussion, Vibration, and Friction.*—
With the edge of the hands percussion is applied
from the forehead and backward to the neck,
three to five times. Then a rapid percussion is
given alternately, with the finger-tips of both
hands, all over the forehead and temples, the
crown of the head, and the neck, four to eight
times. Then one hand is placed on the patient's
forehead and the other is pressed with the inner
edge on the neck just below the base of the skull,
and shaken in a very rapid manner. Repeated
three to five times.

Now a circular and vibratory friction is applied
with the finger-tips several times over the forehead and temples and backward to the neck,
finished up with straight frictions by both hands
and fingers from the middle of the forehead out
to both sides, and backward and down the neck.

These movements are very useful in cases of
headache, weariness, insomnia, etc.

60. *Head Rotation—Sitting.*—The operator
places his one hand on the patient's neck, and
the other hand on his forehead, and slowly moves

the head in a circle, five to ten times one way, then as many times the other way.

This acts on the blood-vessels and nerves of the neck and throat; it is a derivative movement from the brain, and has a quieting effect.

B. *Resistive Movements.*

61. *Neck Flexion and Extension—Standing or Sitting.*—The operator places his one hand on the back of the patient's skull and resists him when he bends his head backward as far as possible. Repeated five to ten times.

This acts on the muscles of the neck and the upper part of the back and on the blood-vessels and nerves of the neck and throat. It is derivative from the brain, and it tends to straighten the upper part of the spine.

Can the Human Hand Be Substituted for Apparatus?

On this head the following from Dr. J. Schreiber may be quoted:—

"Many devices have been invented for saving the manipulator's strength, such as Klemm's muscle-beater, the elastic rods with rubber balls of Graham, and the machines run by steam of Zander.

3*

"All these are well enough in their way for treating certain phases of diseases; but, in general, they may be said to be wholly inadequate to our needs, and are quite apt to degenerate into mere playthings. No better results can be obtained than with the practiced hand, which surpasses even the best of instruments, and the skilled operator needs no other aid, no matter what kind of manipulation he may wish to perform. In the fingers, the fist, the edge of the hand, and in the forearm and arm we have an armamentarium possessed of the greatest variety of effects, for their use is capable of infinite multiplication by the variously graded force with which they may be employed. On the other hand, in executing passive and active muscle exercises, apparatus can be used to the advantage of both patient and physician. Indeed, without it, treatment would often be rendered far more difficult. Nevertheless, it is possible to dispense with special apparatus, and, by employing instead such household furniture as may be at hand, still attain one's end and effect a cure.

"The physician will have frequently an opportunity to display on these occasions his ingenuity and intelligence."

The author agrees with the above-mentioned authority in this, although there are many cases where the use of some kind of apparatus would

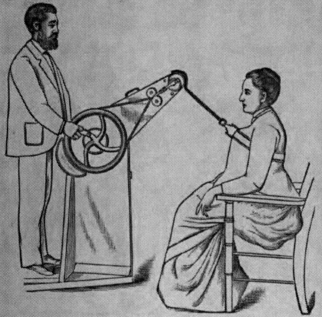

FIG. 28.—THORAX VIBRATION.

greatly hasten the cure and even would be a necessity.

None of all the different movements are so fatiguing to the operator as the *vibrations*, as these must be executed with a great deal of

perseverance and velocity to produce the proper
physiological effect.   There must consequently
be a great advantage in having these movements
executed by machinery.   Such an instrument,

"THE VIBRATOR,"

has been invented by Mr. J. W. Osborne, of

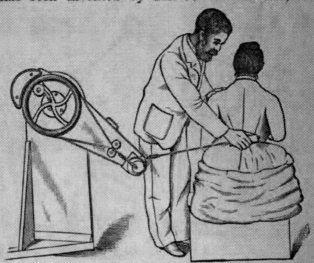

FIG. 29.—BACK VIBRATION.

Washington, D. C., for the use of the author.
It has been used for over three years at his institute in Washington, and has proved a great success in many cases where hardly anything would
have been accomplished without it.

This instrument (Figs. 28, 29) is portable; is constructed and adapted for being brought up to the patient and applied in whatever position it may be desirable to place him, whether standing, sitting, or lying. The rapidity of vibration is subject to very great variations, and may rise from four or five per second to fifty, sixty, or even seventy impulses in the same time. The power of the vibration may be altered so as to suit the strongest as well as the most delicate and feeble person, and the vibration may be applied to any part, muscle, or nerve of the human body.

On tired or aching muscles or nerves the vibratory movements have a very refreshing and soothing effect. Pain is lessened, indeed, is very often entirely subdued, by a single vibration lasting only a few minutes.

On the other hand, a truly physiological stimulation of a nerve may be effected the intensity of which may be easily controlled.

When a percussive vibration is given on the os sacrum, the patient can easily feel the walls of the rectum and bladder contract.

Vibration, applied to the ear and surrounding tissues, or to the nose and larynx, stimulates the nerves (or the parts), thus increasing the circula-

tion of the blood, whereby the mucous membrane
function is facilitated; the feeling of heat and
pressure disappears; respiration is easier; the
uneasy, burning sensation in the throat and in
catarrh of the larynx is relieved, and the voice
will be clearer.

Vibration of the chest (the thorax vibration)
has a *specific action* not only on respiration, but
on the *heart* also. Its contractions become less
frequent but more effective.

In many cases its effect on the respiration is
remarkable. In several instances the number
of respirations per minute have been reduced
from thirty-four to twenty-two, with a single application of half a minute's duration.

Slow vibration of the heavy muscles and vis-
cera are most effective in promoting the venous
circulation in such organs, and therefore their
nutrition and elimination of effete matter.

Fig. 28 shows the machine in position to
apply "thorax vibration."

Fig. 29 shows the "back vibration."

CHAPTER IV.

GROUP I.

CONSTITUTIONAL DISEASES.

A. CHLOROSIS AND ANÆMIA, NEURASTHENIA, HYSTERIA, AND HYPOCHONDRIA.

THE character of these diseases is weakness, therefore it may seem strange to treat them with movements. To apply fatiguing movements would also be as absurd as to prescribe weakening medicines, but by stimulating and strengthening movements re-establishment may be accomplished.

Dr. J. Schreiber says: "For the treatment of this group of diseases, considered as a whole, the following physiological principles should be kept in mind:—

"The muscles being the chief site of chemical change occurring in the body, stimulating and

(63)

increasing their action leads to increased oxygenation of the blood; to greater combustion of
oxygen and elimination of carbonic acid; to increased metabolism and consequently to greater
desire for food and to better digestion; to produc-
tion of more and better blood; to improved nour-
ishment of the nervous system; to an increase,
both in number and strength, of the muscle-
fibres; to the endowment of the whole body
with vigor and elasticity, and to a consequent
revival of all the mental faculties."

Although these are the principles of treatment,
the prescription of movements in each of these
diseases will require considerable variation.

"*In chlorosis and anæmia* the blood-vessels
are both thin-walled and of narrow calibre;
therefore, active and resistive movements should
be used, which stimulates cardiac activity and
increases the blood pressure. The augmented
hæmic oxygenation thus brought about leads
both to an increase in the number of red corpus-
cles as well as of the amount of hæmoglobin
contained in each. At first, owing to the general
lassitude from which chlorotics suffer, the movements will have to be of a very gentle nature."

Although there may be a little difference in

the treatment of two different persons, it should always be directed so as to restore the digestion, circulation, and respiration.

In the first two or three weeks the following prescription would be most acceptable.

Prescription I.

1. Shoulder rotation and chest lifting—sitting.
2. Foot rotation—double—reclining.
3. Stomach vibration—reclining—knees bent.
4. Forward arm rotation—sitting.
5. Trunk rotation—astride sitting.
6. Knee flexion and extension—sitting—resistive.
7. Stomach friction—lying.
8. Back percussion and friction.

The first movement is a respiratory one; the chest is expanded, the inspiration becomes deeper and is followed by a stronger expiration. Thus a greater amount of oxygen is taken and waste matter given off. This must stimulate the functions of the organs and thus accelerate the process of renewal and an exchange of material in all parts of the body.

The second movement equalizes the circulation by increasing the flow of blood to the feet.

The third movement has a direct effect on the stomach, and will improve the appetite and the digestion.

The fourth movement is a respiratory one and has a similar effect as the first one.

The fifth movement brings the muscles of the waist and bowels into play, and acts on the circulation, especially in the portal system.

The sixth movement has a strengthening effect on the flexors and extensors of the legs and promotes the circulation.

The seventh movement promotes operations of the bowels.

The eighth movement has a stimulating effect on the nerve-centres.

When the prescription has been applied for a while, and the patient has improved in strength, the treatment may be changed in force, but according to the same principle.

Prescription II.

1. Forward trunk flexion and extension—sitting—resistive.

2. Foot flexion and extension—double—reclining—resistive.

3. Trunk torsion—sitting—resistive.

4. Vertical arm flexion and extension—sitting.

5. Forward trunk elevation—lying—active.

6. Leg flexion and extension—reclining—resistive.

7. Stomach friction—lying.

8. Breech beating—standing.

9. Back percussion and friction—standing.

"In the treatment of *neurasthenia* and its allied affections, *hysteria* and *hypochondria*, we seek to attain a three-fold end: First, to regenerate the mass of blood as a whole; secondly, to combat individual symptoms; and, thirdly, to favorably influence the mental state.

"Beard, who claims for neurasthenia that it is a new, and especially American disease, considers movement treatment as not only essential, but absolutely indispensable for those cases which it seems advisable to confine in bed." (Dr. J. Schreiber.)

Dr. Weir Mitchell says, in his "Fat and Blood," that he has applied massage *to deprive rest of its evils.*

Amid all the numerous morbid manipulations accompanying neurasthenia, hyperæsthesia and muscular weakness are probably the most prominent, so that Arndt has declared the nature of

the disease to consist in *increased irritability,
with rapid tendency to fatigue, especially of the
muscular system.*

In neurasthenia, all the morbid processes occurring in the muscles are more rapidly influ-
enced by movement treatment than by either
hydro- or electro- therapy. Of all symptoms the
various hyperæsthesias most frequently engage
the physician's attention.

These are generally regarded by the friends as
founded either on exaggeration or upon affectation.
Patients complain of muscular pains, especially
in the extremities and back, and of pains along
the spinal column, the latter being, indeed, considered quite characteristic of the disease ("spinal
irritation").

Besides these, neurasthenics suffer from the
greatest variety of symptoms referable to the
brain, as headache, and a feeling of weight or
constriction in the head, eye, and ear, photopsia,
scotoma, roaring and ringing in the ears, hyper-
sensitiveness to odors, and other similar idiosyn-
crasies. Or there may be liability to sudden
changes of temper, or to depression and sadness,
or dizziness or insomnia may exist. Indeed, the
large number of various feelings of apprehension

experienced in neurasthenia has been the occasion for the manufacture, by various authors, of any number of "phobias." The restlessness so often seen in these patients is caused by the pains occurring in various muscle groups.

The so-called "general massage" of the whole body will be found the most effectual in banishing the various anæsthesias and hyperæsthesias, while passive rotation, flexion, and extension cause a stretching of the nerves contained within the muscles, which reacts most favorably upon the mental state.

Prescription I.

1. Legs—centripetal stroking, pressing, kneading, circular and vibratory friction.

2. Arms—centripetal stroking, pressing, kneading, circular and vibratory friction.

3. Chest kneading and friction.

4. Stomach kneading and friction.

5. Back kneading and friction.

6. Head friction.

This treatment should be applied daily, and even twice a day, until the patient has gained some strength.

Advisable to increase the treatment, as in the following:—

Prescription II.

1. Legs — centripetal stroking, pressing, kneading, circular and vibratory friction.

2. Foot rotation—single.

3. Thigh rotation.

4. Arms— centripetal stroking, pressing, kneading, circular and vibratory friction.

5. Hand, forearm, and arm rotation.

6. Chest lifting and vibration.

7. Chest kneading, slapping, and friction.

8. Stomach kneading, vibration, and friction.

9. Arms—nerve compression, rolling, slapping, and friction.

10. Legs—nerve compression, rolling, slapping, and friction.

11. Back kneading, percussion, and friction.

12. Head percussion, kneading, and friction.

All these different movements must, of course, be applied with great care and gentleness in the beginning, but by degrees the force may be increased until the patient no longer is confined to the bed, when the movements should be changed to

Prescription III.

1. Forward arm rotation—sitting—passive.

2. Foot rotation—double—reclining—passive.

3. Trunk rotation—astride sitting—passive.

4. Vertical arm flexion and extension—sitting —resistive.

5. Leg flexion and extension—reclining—resistive.

6. Chest slapping—standing—passive.

7. Arm—nerve compression, rolling, slapping, and friction—reclining.

8. Leg—nerve compression, rolling, slapping, and friction—reclining.

9. Stomach kneading, vibration, and friction.

10. Back percussion and friction—standing.

11. Head percussion, kneading, and friction— sitting.

Hysteria and hypochondria are, according to Arndt, quite impossible to separate from neurasthenia. He considered the numerous terms of different authors—such as spinal neurosis, spasmophilia, spinal weakness or irritability, nervosism, eretheism, and others—to be but different names for one and the same condition. The different writers seem, however, to be of the opinion that it is impossible to permanently cure this condition, and that no medicaments exist capable of permanently allaying the irritability of the hyperæsthetic nerves.

Nevertheless, a daily course of carefully system-
atized exercise will always be of great value to
these patients, and they, therefore, ought to be
recommended to some establishment where movement treatment is a specialty.

B. INSOMNIA.

Of the numerous cases of insomnia which have
come under the writer's observation, the following described one was considered by the attending physicians to be exceedingly dangerous, and
one in which the patient was so weak and irritable that the greatest care and gentleness were
imperative.

The 1st of October, 1887, the writer was
called to see a gentleman, forty years old, who
had been without sleep for three weeks. He was
very weak and complained of great pain in the
back, legs, and wrists. He was very nervous and
irritable, and had no appetite.

The first two days only the following movements were applied :—

1. Arms—friction—downward.
2. Legs—friction—downward.
3. Back friction—downward.
4. Head friction.

The patient had some sleep the first night, which was increased a little every following night.

The third day the treatment was increased as follows :—

1. Arms — nerve compression, rolling, and friction.

2. Legs—nerve compression, rolling, and friction.

3. Chest friction.

4. Stomach friction.

5. Back kneading and friction.

6. Head kneading and friction.

The force of the manipulation was increased a little every day.

· The seventh day the following treatment was applied :—

1. Legs—thigh rotation.

2. Arms—arm rotation and hand rotation.

3. Chest lifting and vibration.

4. Chest slapping, kneading, and friction.

5. Stomach kneading and friction.

6. Arms — nerve compression, rolling, and friction.

7. Legs—nerve compression, rolling, and friction.

8. Back kneading, vibration, percussion, and friction.

9. Head percussion, kneading, and friction.

After two weeks' treatment the patient slept the whole night, and he did not complain of any pains, and accordingly resistive movements were added to the former ones in the following manner:—

1. Legs—foot rotation, double—passive.

2. Arms—rotation and hand rotation—passive.

3. Chest lifting and vibration.

4. Chest slapping, kneading, and friction.

5. Stomach kneading and friction.

6. Arms—flexion and extension—resistive.

7. Arms—nerve compression, rolling, slapping, and friction.

8. Legs—flexion and extension—resistive.

9. Legs—nerve compression, rolling, slapping, and friction.

10. Back kneading, vibration, percussion, and friction.

11. Head rotation—sitting.

12. Head percussion, kneading, and friction.

One month after the treatment began the patient was well.

GROUP II.

LOCAL DISEASES.—DISEASES OF THE BRAIN, SPINAL
CORD, AND NERVES.

CONGESTION OF THE BRAIN (CONGESTIO CEREBRALIS).

Severe acute congestion of the brain will
hardly be favorable to movement treatment, but
milder cases have often been treated with success.
The movements should be directed so as to derive
the blood from the brain, therefore movements of
the extremities and the bowels should be applied.
If the patient is not confined to bed the following prescription would be useful:—

1. Shoulder rotation and chest lifting—sitting.
2. Thigh rotation—reclining.
3. Trunk rotation—astride sitting.
4. Leg flexion and extension—reclining—resistive.
5. Neck flexion and extension—standing—
resistive.
6. Foot rotation and flexion and extension—
double—reclining.
7. Forward arm rotation—sitting.
8. Breech beating—standing.
9. Stomach kneading and friction—reclining.

10. Knee flexion and extension—sitting—resistive.

11. Head percussion, vibration, and friction.

ANÆMIA OF THE BRAIN.

The movements in these cases should be stimulating and strengthening.

1. Chest lifting and vibration—lying.

2. Leg nerve compression, rolling, slapping, and friction.

3. Arm compression, rolling, slapping, and friction.

4. Head rotation—sitting.

5. Leg vibration—lying.

6. Arm vibration—sitting.

7. Stomach friction—lying.

8. Back percussion and friction.

9. Head percussion, kneading, vibration, and friction.

PARALYSIS AS A RESULT OF APOPLEXY.

The treatment here is to avoid new attacks as well as to improve the patient's condition, and for this reason the movements should not only be applied to the paralyzed arm and leg, but to the whole body.

The following illustration of this mode of treatment gives the best example of prescriptions for such patients:—

A gentleman, sixty-four years old, was stricken with apoplexy, resulting in a partial paralysis of the right side. Forty-eight hours later the writer was called in by his physician to try the movement treatment. The patient was at this time still unconscious.

The first day the following movements were applied very gently:—

1. Right arm nerve compression and friction.
2. Right hand and finger rotation.
3. Right leg nerve compression and friction.
4. Right foot rotation.
5. Right leg muscle rolling and friction.
6. Right arm muscle rolling and friction.

The next day the patient seemed to know what was going on, as he saw the operator and objected to have a stranger about him. Nevertheless, by kind words and cheerfulness, he consented to the treatment. There was now a slight movement of the right leg, and there was applied, in addition to the former prescription:—

Thigh rotation and *leg flexion and extension, passive*, to the right leg.

The third day the patient was glad to see the operator and delighted to show him his improvement, as he now was able to draw his knee up, make a slight motion of the foot, and of the arm.

His right hand and fingers were swollen and painful, and he could not see with his right eye, and he spoke with difficulty.

Centripetal stroking and kneading was first applied to the right fingers, hand, and arm, together with the following movements:—

Right hand and finger rotation and flexion—passive;

Right arm rotation and flexion—passive;

Centripetal stroking and kneading of right leg;

Right foot rotation and flexion—passive;

Thigh rotation and leg flexion—both legs—passive;

Both arms—nerve compression, rolling, and friction;

Both legs—nerve compression, rolling, and friction.

The fourth day no treatment was given.

The fifth day considerable improvement was noticed in moving both the arm and leg; the swelling and pain of the right hand were very much less. The same movements were used as at the last time.

The sixth day no treatment was applied.

The seventh day the improvement was astonishing, the swelling of the right hand had disappeared, and the patient was able to take me by the hand and to move his foot and leg at will. Prescription was then changed to the following:—

Chest lifting and vibration;

Thigh rotation of both legs;

Right arm rotation;

Foot rotation, double;

Right hand and finger rotation and flexion—passive;

Right leg nerve compression, rolling, and friction;

Right arm nerve compression, rolling, and friction;

Right leg vibration;

Right arm vibration;

Back kneading, percussion, and friction.

This treatment was repeated the eighth, tenth, and eleventh days after the first visit.

The twelfth day the patient was up and able to walk a little in his room, and the following prescription was then given:—

Shoulder rotation and chest lifting—sitting;

Thigh rotation, both legs—reclining;

Right arm rotation—sitting;

Right foot flexion and extension—sitting—resistive;

Right arm nerve compression, rolling, slapping, and friction;

Right leg nerve compression, rolling, slapping, and friction;

Right arm flexion and extension—resistive;

Forward trunk flexion and extension—sitting —resistive;

Right knee flexion and extension—sitting— resistive;

Right arm torsion—resistive;

Right arm vibration—sitting;

Trunk rotation—astride sitting—passive;

Right leg torsion—resistive;

Right leg vibration—reclining;

Back percussion and friction—standing;

Head kneading and friction.

The improvement continued from day to day. The eyesight came back, the speech was clearer, and the patient gained more and more control over his limbs. The treatment was continued every other day for two weeks more, when the patient commenced to take out-door walks.

The fifth week only two treatments were applied and then entirely discontinued, the patient being able to walk as well as before the stroke, and having full use of his arm.

This case was a very favorable one, but there can be no doubt that the movement treatment hastened the improvement considerably, although the physician must be careful not to apply this treatment too soon, and that it is done in a very gentle and judicious manner.

When the physician does not feel sure that the movements will have a good effect it will always be best to wait from four to six weeks before they are resorted to.

The most cases of paralysis are slow to recover, and especially is the hand, as a rule, far behind the rest of the body in becoming well. The treatment is agreeable to this kind of patients and it has a soothing and cheerful influence on them.

Here it may be well to say that all persons who have been troubled once with apoplexy ought never to stop taking movement treatment, or at least only at short intervals, unless they have plenty of other healthful exercise, as it is the best means to prevent another stroke.

CONGESTION OF THE SPINE.

This disease has often been quickly improved by a proper treatment of derivative movements, which are herein set forth :—

1. Forward arm rotation—sitting—passive.
2. Foot rotation, double—reclining—passive.
3. Vertical arm flexion and extension—sitting—resistive.
4. Leg flexion and extension—reclining—resistive.
5. Trunk torsion—astride sitting—resistive.
6. Bent knee separation and closing—reclining—resistive.
7. Breech beating—standing—passive.
8. Knee flexion and extension—sitting—resistive.
9. Stomach friction—lying—passive.
10. Shoulder rotation and chest lifting—sitting.

SCIATIC NEURALGIA.

Of all writers on the treatment of this malady Dr. J. Schreiber seems to have had the most experience and to have been the most successful in his cures. Upon this subject he says :—

" As the greater number of sciaticas which
have come under my notice have been combined
with crural neuralgia as well, I think it best to
consider these two conditions together. It seems
advisable, also, to discuss the treatment according
to a plan which may, with suitable modifications,
be applied to each special case, and yet one which
will embrace the details gleaned from numerous
observations. Let us take a case :—

" A patient suffering from well-marked sciatica
and crural neuralgia of the right side applies for
relief, after having been under treatment by others
for many years in vain. He has used veratria,
aconite, and belladonna ointments, morphine in-
jections, electricity, sinapisms, and vesicants. We
may assume, also, that for a considerable period
he took arsenic, quinine, and potassium iodide
and bromide, that he has been to a number of
springs, like Gastein, Wiesbaden, Teplitz, and
Ragaz, and also that neither sea-bathing nor
hydrotherapy has had any effect upon his obsti-
nate malady. He is only able to drag himself
painfully along by the use of a cane, and every
step causes acute suffering. Rising and sitting
down can only be accomplished by aid of the
arms, while for going up stairs or getting out of

bed the assistance of an attendant is necessary. He is never entirely free from pain, and there is generally a daily exacerbation lasting often several hours, and preventing much-needed rest.

"Examination shows no other functional disturbances. There is great sensitiveness in the buttock, at the point of exit of the sciatic nerve, and many painful points exist along the outer and inner aspects of the thigh. The limb, furthermore, will be seen to be held in a characteristically pathognomonic position, namely, the thigh rotated inward and adducted, the knee slightly bent, and the foot not resting on the ground with the sole, but touching it with the toe only.

"On sitting down, the patient supports himself by his left arm, and lets himself fall, as it were, upon his left buttock, instead of performing the usual movements of flexion with knees and hips. The involvement of the semitendinosus and semimembranosus muscles causes great sensitiveness to pressure over their tendons. Voluntary abduction of the affected thigh is impossible, and abduction of even the well extremity cannot be performed on standing erect, on account of inability of the patient to support himself upon the affected limb. External rotation is also impossible. Hence it appears that the glutei, the pyriformis, the internal obturator, and the gemelli (external rotators) are all affected. Nor can the patient flex the thigh (involvement of the iliac and psoas major), nor can he adduct it after it has once been passively abducted (involvement of the sartorius, internal rectus, adductors longus, brevis and magnus, and pectineus). But the greatest pain of all is caused by rotating the thigh outward, as the sciatic is thus made to glide upon and rub against the quadratus femoris.

" I have purposely selected a case in which all the muscles of the buttock, about the hip-joint, and of the thigh have become involved, and hence almost entirely deprived of function. Many years of experience and many trials have convinced me that the cure of these forms of sciatica will be most rapidly effected when, in addition to the mechanical interferences, passive and active motions of all the affected muscles are employed. It has also seemed to me best to begin the daily treatment with the passive and active movements, leaving the mechanical manipulations, which are very painful, till the last. They cause so much exhaustion, as a rule, that the patient is anxious only for rest, and will hardly have the energy necessary for performing acts which he knows must only increase his suffering."

If the cause of the neuralgia is a pressure, as from a tumor, etc., it is of no use to try this treatment, but otherwise it will generally effect a cure. At the end of each day's treatment the patient will generally complain of much pain and fatigue, which usually diminishes considerably in about half an hour, although it sometimes lasts for hours afterward. In the beginning, too, the night's rest may be more broken than before. In six to twelve days usually a change for the better occurs, the night's rest becoming more tranquil, the pain less, and the first signs of approaching convalescence begin to appear.

Dr. Schreiber says: "It is almost a matter of course that the physician will be confronted with every kind of doubt on the part of the patient regarding the ultimate results of treatment, but, as failures are rare where sufficient perseverance and the requisite skill have been employed, he may confidently combat these misapprehensions. The duration of the treatment will depend on the following various factors:—

"1. On the previous length of the illness.

" The longer the disease has existed the more protracted will have to be the treatment. Eight weeks will, as a rule, be the limit; at least, that was the limit needed to cure one of my cases of a previous four years' duration. Cases of only a few months' standing often need but ten or twelve days for a cure.

" 2. On the extent of the disease.

" The greater the number of muscles involved the more numerous must the number of corresponding exercises be, and hence the longer the time required.

" 3. On idiosyncrasy.

" In sensitive individuals it is often necessary to proceed very cautiously and gently at first. More time is, therefore, required in these cases than where the patient is not of a timorous or complaining disposition.

" 4. On the skill, the experience, and the perseverance of the physician.

" Familiarity with the methods frequently enables a practiced hand to employ many devices which an inexperienced person very properly avoids.

" 5. On the age and general nutrition of the patient."

Two very interesting cases are illustrated by Dr. Schreiber, and he claims to have cured numerous persons of very bad sciatica. His mode of treatment is in its character the same as the writer has been using, but as Dr. Schreiber already, the first day of treatment, uses some kind of apparatus, the description below given shows the method found by the writer to be the best where the patient is confined to his room, as in a case of sciatica of the right leg.

The first day the treatment must be very gentle and of short duration, the patient lying down.

1. Right leg flexion and extension—passive—four to ten times, according to his strength.

2. Right leg nerve compression and rolling.

3. Breech beating.

4. Right leg (back of the thigh) percussion and friction.

The second day the same treatment with more force.

The third day the following is applied:—

1. Right leg flexion and extension—passive.

2. Right leg nerve compression and rolling.

3. Right thigh rotation.

4. Right leg vibration.

5. Breech beating.

6. Right leg nerve compression, percussion, and friction.

The fourth day give:—

1. Right thigh rotation.
2. Right leg flexion and extension—resistive.
3. Right leg nerve compression and rolling.
4. Right leg separation and closing—passive.
5. Right foot flexion and extension—resistive.
6. Right leg vibration.
7. Breech beating.
8. Right leg nerve compression, percussion, and friction.

The fifth, sixth, and seventh days we may apply deep kneading of all the muscles of the buttock and thigh, just before "breech beating," in connection with the former prescription.

The next four or five days the following movements should be used:—

1. Thigh rotation—both legs—passive.
2. Right leg flexion and extension—resistive.
3. Right leg nerve compression and rolling.
4. Right leg torsion—passive.
5. Right leg separation and closing—resistive.
6. Kneading and beating of right leg and buttock
7. Right knee upward traction—resistive.

D*

8. Right foot flexion and extension—resistive.

9. Right leg vibration.

10. Right leg nerve compression, rolling, and friction.

The last prescription, which may be continued till the patient is well, has a more all-sided effect.

1. Thigh rotation—both legs—passive.

2. Right leg nerve compression, rolling, and friction.

3. Trunk rotation—astride sitting—passive.

4. Right leg flexion and extension—resistive.

5. Kneading and beating of right leg and buttock.

6. Forward trunk flexion and extension—sitting—resistive.

7. Bent knee separation and closing—resistive.

8. Right leg percussion.

9. Right leg torsion—resistive.

10. Breech beating.

11. Foot rotation, double—passive.

12. Right leg nerve compression, rolling, and friction.

In connection with this, it will be of great advantage to let the patient walk and run on tiptoe, and to go up and down a few steps, or stairs.

There should also be taken good care that the patient always sits straight and rests evenly on both buttocks.

Of the many cases of sciatica which the writer has treated, the following one was cured in the shortest time, considering the previous duration of the disease :—

A lady, twenty-nine years old, suffered from sciatica for ten months. She had been in bed most of the time, and all kinds of treatment had been tried without any relief. One day, in August, 1885, she felt well enough to be taken in a carriage and carried into the writer's Institute, where the movement treatment was applied. It pained her a great deal, but after awhile it gave her relief, and she returned the next day. The fifth day she walked alone to the Institute, and after three weeks' treatment was cured. She has not had any return of the disease since.

In this case the "vibrator" was used in connection with the other movements, giving a "tractional" vibration to the whole leg and a "percussive" vibration on the sciatic nerve, which has been found to be of a very great value.

FOR WRITER'S CRAMP.

These movements are useful:—

1. Back percussion.
2. Right arm centripetal stroking, pressing, kneading, circulatory and vibratory friction.
3. Right arm rotation.
4. Forward trunk flexion and extension—sitting—resistive.
5. Right arm torsion—resistive.
6. Right hand and finger flexion and extension—resistive.
7. Right arm vibration.
8. Trunk rotation—astride sitting—passive.
9. Vertical arm flexion and extension—resistive.
10. Right arm nerve compression, rolling, slapping, and friction.

CRAMP OF THE LEGS.

1. Thigh rotation.
2. Leg vibration.
3. Foot flexion and extension—resistive.
4. Trunk torsion—sitting—resistive.
5. Leg nerve compression, rolling, and friction.

6. Leg flexion and extension—resistive.

7. Trunk elevation—lying—active.

8. Upward knee traction—resistive.

9. Breech beating.

10. Leg torsion—resistive.

11. Leg nerve compression, slapping, and friction.

12. Back percussion and friction.

CHOREA.

This disease has been treated with great success by the Swedish movement.

M. Napoleon Laisné has applied this treatment to hundreds of children at the "Hôpital des Enfants Malades," in Paris, with the greatest success. Dr. Blache, the president of this hospital, addressed in 1851 an assembly of directors and prominent physicians upon the results of this treatment. He closed his report by saying that in four years not one of the choreic children thus treated had suffered a relapse.

Both active, resistive, and passive movements should be used; but, as these cases require a great deal of patience and an experienced gymnast to lead them on, no prescription for this treatment is given here.

GROUP III.

DISEASES OF THE ORGANS OF THE CIRCULATION.
CHRONIC HEART DISEASES.

In these cases movements must be given which shall diminish the pressure of the blood and decrease the activity of the heart.

Inspiration acts as a pump on the circulation toward the heart. Muscle-contractions produce a pressure on the walls of the blood-vessels, whereby the blood is forced toward the heart; hence, respiratory and circulatory movements are here of great value.

Dr. Gustaf Zander, of the Mechanico-Therapeutic Institute in Stockholm, says: "In heart diseases, movement treatment is an uninterrupted necessity, at least during the winter. It is a pity when in such cases the patients have no opportunity to use this treatment. It is astonishing what excellent effects regular, gentle, but many-sided muscular exercises have on diseases of the heart. Some of these, when not too far gone, can be entirely cured, others can be stopped from further development, and all can be relieved."

From Dr. Hartelius, the Principal of the Royal Central Gymnastic Institute, in Stockholm, we quote the following:—

"A lady, thirty years old, with a dangerous organic heart disease—*stenosis of left ostium atrioventriculare, with insufficiency of mitralis.* The action of the heart was very weak. The patient suffered with great shortness of breath and painful palpitations; a great deal of subcutaneous effusion in the lower extremities and also considerable effusion in the peritoneum. Her aspect was cyanotical.

"*Mild chest liftings and vibrations* were given to produce strong inspirations, also *rotation* of the arms and legs to increase the circulation, gentle *rotation* and torsion of the trunk to act on the portal system, and centripetal friction on the lower extremities to promote resorption of the subcutaneous effusion. In the beginning the movements were very mild, but gave relief for a few hours at a time. Later the movements were applied several times daily, and then more lasting effects were produced. Patient received great relief, more strength, and the effusion was lessened, but her organic trouble could not be cured.

"Experience tells us that each difficult heart disease must nearly always be under the influence of movement treatment in order to secure permanently good results."

After this, it will be understood that the most advisable thing for those suffering to do is to go to a specialist who has the most experience in their treatment.

Still, there are many cases where the patient is too weak to go out, and he may receive great relief in his room by the following:—

1. Chest lifting and vibration.

2. Foot rotation, double.

3. Arms — centripetal stroking, pressing, kneading, and friction.

4. Legs—centripetal stroking, pressing, kneading, and friction.

5. Hand and finger rotation, flexion, and extension—passive.

6. Thigh rotation.

7. Chest percussion.

8. Loin traction.

9. Leg vibration.

10. Back percussion and friction.

FOR COLD HANDS AND FEET

the following movements are very useful:—

1. Forward arm rotation—sitting—passive.

2. Foot rotation, double—reclining—passive.

3. Vertical arm flexion and extension—sitting—resistive.

4. Leg flexion and extension—reclining—resistive.

5. Trunk rotation—astride—passive.

6. Hand and finger flexion and extension—resistive.

7. Foot flexion and extension—resistive.

8. Arm nerve compression, rolling, slapping, and friction.

9. Leg nerve compression, rolling, slapping, and friction.

10. Arm vibration.

11. Foot-sole slapping and friction.

12. Back percussion and friction.

GROUP IV.

DISEASES OF THE RESPIRATORY ORGANS.

Catarrh of the larynx, catarrh of the lungs, congestion of the lungs, emphysema of the lungs, spasmus bronchialis, and even *tuberculosis* have all been treated with success at different establishments by movements, but each of them requires quite a special treatment by a skillful and experienced gymnast, and, therefore, only a prescription for movements to be used where there is a disposition to a lung trouble, showing a narrow chest, round and stooping shoulders, and lack of muscular power, is here given:—

1. Shoulder rotation and chest lifting—sitting.

2. Foot flexion and extension—resistive.

3. Trunk torsion—sitting—resistive.

4. Forward arm rotation—sitting.

5. Leg flexion and extension—reclining—resistive.

6. Horizontal arm separation and closing—resistive.

7. Neck flexion and extension—standing—resistive.

8. Forward trunk flexion and extension—sitting—resistive.

9. Lateral arm elevation and depression—sitting—resistive.

10. Chest slapping.

GROUP V.

DISEASES OF THE ORGANS OF DIGESTION.

The following prescriptions are given only for the most frequent cases, as *dyspepsia, constipation,* and *hyperæmia of the liver.* The treatment in these cases should be directed to strengthen the whole system, as well as to act locally on the diseased organ.

DYSPEPSIA.

If the patient is very weak it will be necessary to give him a light treatment for the first two or three weeks, viz.:—

1. Arm nerve compression, rolling, slapping, and friction.
2. Legs the same.
3. Stomach vibration and friction.
4. Thigh rotation.
5. Arm vibration.
6. Chest lifting and vibration.
7. Stomach kneading and friction.
8. Leg vibration.
9. Back percussion and friction.

When the patient is improved and has gained some strength, not confined to bed, the following should be applied:—

1. Forward arm rotation—sitting—passive.
2. Stomach kneading, vibration, and friction.
3. Upward knee traction—reclining—resistive.
4. Trunk rotation—astride sitting—passive.
5. Stomach concussion and friction—lying.
6. Leg elevation—lying—resistive.

7. Vertical arm flexion and extension — resistive.

8. Loin traction—lying.

9. Leg flexion and extension — reclining — resistive.

10. Back percussion and friction.

CONSTIPATION.

If the patient is in bed a local manipulation for about five to ten minutes twice a day will be most effective, viz.:—

1. Stomach kneading, vibration, concussion, and friction—five to ten minutes.

2. Breech beating.

3. Loin traction.

If the disease is of long standing it is necessary to apply strong muscular movements, as :—

1. Forward trunk flexion and extension—sitting—resistive.

2. Upward knee traction—reclining—resistive.

3. Bowel vibration—standing—passive.

4. Trunk elevation—lying—active.

5. Trunk rotation—astride sitting—passive.

6. Stomach kneading and friction—reclining.

7. Trunk torsion—kneeling—resistive.

8. Vertical arm flexion and extension—lying—resistive.

9. Loin vibration—sitting—passive.

10. Breech beating—standing—passive.

11. Stomach kneading, concussion, and friction.

12. Shoulder rotation and chest lifting — sitting—passive.

HYPERÆMIA OF THE LIVER.

The following cited case of this disease will be especially interesting :—

A gentleman of middle age had been ailing two years. He had grown very lean, the skin was yellow, and his feet and ankles were swollen. The liver was considerably enlarged, especially the left lobe. There was no organic heart disease, but there was a mild catarrh of the lungs. Operations of the bowels were slow and difficult. He was treated twice every day by means of movements, and no other remedies were used. After one month the patient was considerably better, the liver was smaller, swelling had disappeared, and his appetite and flesh had increased. After the second month, having been treated once a day, the patient was cured.

The following prescription was used :—

1. Shoulder rotation and chest lifting—sitting.

2. Foot rotation, double—reclining.

3. Trunk rotation—astride sitting.

4. Vertical arm flexion and extension—resistive.

5. Loin vibration—sitting.

6. Thigh rotation—reclining.

7. Chest lifting and vibration—reclining.

8. Leg flexion and extension—reclining—resistive.

9. Stomach kneading and friction—reclining.

10. Back percussion and friction—standing.

GROUP VI.

DISEASES OF URINARY AND SEXUAL ORGANS.

CHRONIC CATARRH OF THE BLADDER.

The movements should be derivative from the pelvis and otherwise be directed according to the patient's condition—for instance :—

1. Thigh rotation—reclining.

2. Breech beating—standing.

3. Bent knee separation and closing—resistive.

4. Forward trunk flexion and extension—sitting—resistive.

5. Leg torsion, double—reclining—resistive.

6. Breech beating—standing.

7. Lateral arm elevation and depression — standing—resistive.

8. Foot rotation, double—reclining.

CHRONIC CATARRH OF THE WOMB.

1. Back percussion and friction—standing.

2. Breech beating—standing.

3. Leg separation and closing — reclining— resistive.

4. Forward arm rotation—sitting.

5. Trunk rotation—astride sitting.

6. Knee flexion and extension—reclining— resistive.

7. Forward trunk flexion and extension— sitting—resistive.

8. Breech beating—standing.

9. Trunk torsion—kneeling—resistive.

10. Back percussion and friction — standing.

Displacement of the womb as well as *irregularity and painful menstruation* are often not only relieved but even cured by movement treatment, but these cases require a special study and experience.

GROUP VII.

DISEASES OF THE ORGANS OF MOVEMENTS.

SCOLIOSIS.

In "*lateral curvature of the spine*," where the muscles on the convex side are weakened and pathologically changed, and the muscles on the concave side normal, it is clear that the weakened muscles on the convex side must be strengthened and developed. According to Dr. T. J. Hartelius, "The restoration of a pathologically changed muscle cannot be produced by mechanical extensions, but only by muscular exercise and electricity.

"But," he says, "for the restoration of a curved spine extension is necessary. The question is, therefore, whether this can be effected by the organism's own remedies. This is easy enough to prove. In mild cases of lateral curvature, where there is not yet any deformity in the vertebræ, the spine is straightened at each extension of the back. By flexion to the convex side the spine is not only straightened, but it can be bent so far as to display a curve to the other side. In cases where the deformity of the vertebræ makes a full extension of the spine impossible, it is still possible by its own strength to produce an extension in its highest degree.

"For instance, in a 'forward trunk flexion and extension' the patient stands supported on the thighs and bends forward; when he raises himself up, the operator resists him on the neck. Or, in 'backward trunk flexion' the patient is lying on the front of his legs and raises the back up backward.

"These and a few other active and resistive movements can, better than any other mechanical remedy, straighten out the curved parts."

In a one-sided scoliosis, for instance, with the convexity to the left, "lateral trunk flexion to the left" may be given. The operator puts his hands on the highest point of the curve and resists the patient when he bends down. This can be performed either with the patient sitting, standing, or lying on his right side, the last one being the most powerful and effective. Several other movements are also given with the view and intention of strengthening the muscles on the convex side and straightening out the spine, and should be used according to the strength of the patient and the particular shape of the deformity.

Dr. Schreiber says: "The treatment of scoli-

5*

osis by the Ling system, which has scored some of its greatest successes in this very department, requires, however, quite a special study, and can hardly be carried out without both apparatus and trained assistants."

Dr. M. Eulenberg, in " Die Schwedische Heil-gymnastick," Berlin, 1853, says:—

" Ling's method is the only truly rational therapeutic means for the cure of chronic disturbances of motivity, such as result from spinal curvature, and from pseudo-anchylosis, the phthisical tendency, pigeon-breast, peripheral paralysis, etc.

" Even in cases of paralysis from lesions of the cord, it may still effect a cure where all other measures, undertaken after the original diseases have run their course, will be found useless. Ling's gymnastics have an even greater and more certain effect upon enervation and nutrition than the common form of gymnastic exercises. Spinal (lateral) curvatures, resulting from faulty carriage (in consequence of a preponderance of muscular force on one side of the body), are nowadays never treated by any good orthopædist by any other means than the Swedish system."

Any one who will undertake the treatment of

scoliosis should make it a special study, as it requires great experience, skill, and knowledge to lead it on successfully.

MUSCULAR RHEUMATISM.
A. *Of the Right Arm.*

1. Centripetal stroking, pressing, kneading, circulatory friction, and vibratory friction of right arm.
2. Thigh rotation—reclining.
3. Right arm muscle beating.
4. Trunk rotation—astride sitting.
5. Right arm flexion and extension—resistive.
6. Leg flexion and extension—resistive.
7. Right arm torsion—resistive.
8. The same as No. 1.
9. Back percussion.

B. *Of the Neck.*

1. Forward arm rotation—sitting.
2. Head rotation—sitting.
3. Foot rotation—reclining.
4. Neck percussion—sitting.
5. Horizontal arm separation and closing—resistive.
6. Trunk torsion—kneeling—resistive.
7. Neck flexion and extension—resistive.

8. Knee flexion and extension — sitting — resistive.

9. Centripetal stroking, pressing, kneading, circulatory and vibratory friction of the neck.

10. Back percussion and friction.

C. *Lumbago.*

1. Forward trunk flexion and extension — sitting—resistive.

2. Thigh rotation—reclining—passive.

3. Trunk rotation—astride sitting—passive.

4. Breech beating—standing—passive.

5. Vertical arm flexion and extension—sitting —resistive.

6. Bent knee separation and closing—reclining—resistive.

7. Muscle kneading, percussion, vibration, and friction all over the small of the back and the buttocks.

These three examples show how to arrange the treatment in the different cases of muscular rheumatism. Of course, if the patient is too sick to take the full prescription, we only apply the local treatment until he is able to take the whole, which has in view the increasing of the circulation and giving nutrition to the whole system, as well as to relieve the local disease.

A few interesting cases it may be well to give here :—

On September 24, 1886, a lady, fifty-five years old, came to the writer. She was five feet six inches tall, and weighed two hundred and thirty pounds. She complained of rheumatism in her legs and arms, and could only walk up one flight of stairs, and that with the greatest difficulty. On her arrival she was gasping for breath and sat down to rest for nearly an hour.

Eight weeks later, having taken treatment every day, the lady asked if she might walk up to the top of the Washington Monument (about nine hundred steps). Although knowing that she had improved marvelously and had lost nearly thirty pounds, the writer told her that it would be better not to try it then, because there was no one to carry her down again if she became too tired.

She laughed and said that she had walked up the monument the previous day, looked around for half an hour, and walked down and to her home, about a quarter of a mile distant. She felt very well after it, and had no lameness nor pain.

After ten weeks' treatment the lady was

entirely well, having had no rheumatism for the last five weeks, and her weight was then one hundred and ninety-six pounds. In the summer of 1887 she called to say that she still felt like a young girl, and was going West to live for the rest of her life.

Other cases are as follow :—

A gentleman, thirty-one years old, had suffered with muscular rheumatism in his right shoulder and arm for two weeks. He had not had any relief or sleep for several days when he came to the writer. Five days later he was cured.

Dr. N. N., forty-six years old, had been in bed about three weeks with a very painful lumbago, and was unable to move himself when he sent for the author, in March, 1883.

Movement treatments were applied six times, after which he was out attending to his own business.

A gentleman, forty-two years old, had suffered from lumbago and indigestion for nearly eight months, and had given up all kinds of treatment. In April, 1883, the writer was called in by one of his friends. The patient, who had once been a very strong and healthy laborer, was run down to a thin, very feeble-looking man. He did not believe in the treatment, but he submitted to a trial of it. The first treatment being satisfactory, it was continued every day. The improvement was remarkable. The pain became less and less, and the appetite and strength were increased every day.

After three weeks' treatment the patient had gained twelve pounds, and he was well enough to attend to his business. The treatment was then discontinued.

Half a year later, when he felt some symptoms of the lumbago, he came to the Institute and took one month's treatment. He has been well ever since.

RHEUMATISM OF THE JOINTS.

If the joints are stiff and cannot be moved, local manipulations, as follow, are useful:—

Centripetal stroking, pressing, kneading, beating, and *friction* of the diseased part and surrounding muscles, from ten to twenty minutes, will include the full treatment for some time, and even for months; but when the joint finally responds to the treatment and allows of some motion, it will be most effective to treat it after the following method, given for rheumatism of the right knee:—

1. Centripetal stroking, pressing, kneading, beating, and friction—five minutes.

2. Right leg flexion and extension—resistive.

3. Trunk rotation—astride sitting.

4. Right knee muscle rolling—reclining.

5. Forward arm rotation—sitting.

6. Thigh rotation—both legs—reclining.

7. Trunk elevation—lying—active.

8. Right knee flexion and extension—sitting—resistive.

9. The same as No. 1.

In the first instance the treatment is given to increase the circulation in and around the joint, to promote absorption, and to squeeze exudations out of the joint.

In the second instance the treatment tends to tone up the whole system by strengthening the circulation and digestive organs.

STIFFNESS OF JOINTS AND TENDONS.

From Dr. Schreiber the following is quoted:—

"It not infrequently happens that, after arthritis, thickening of the periarthritic structures or even adhesion of the articular surfaces themselves may occur, leading to very considerable disability of motions. Only by mechanical means .can we then hope to break up the existing adhesions, to smooth the roughened articular cartilages, and to restore to the ligaments their former suppleness and elasticity.

"All the mechanical interferences used—pressing, stroking, kneading—as well as the passive exercises—must be performed with the greatest care, since it is quite possible to initiate fresh inflammatory action by injudicious treatment.

"The successful treatment of these cases affords one of the most difficult problems of the mechano-thereopist, for it requires untiring perseverance and patience, as well as nice judgment and all the fruits gained by experience, to tide the patient over the necessary pain which for months he may be called upon to bear.

"The *modus operandi* in each case will be indicated by the mechanism of the particular joint to be treated, which sometimes will be found to be immovably fixed.   At first the tissues surrounding the joint are to be gently rubbed, using in the beginning the finger-tips only; later, the force may be increased.

"As soon as the part has, in a measure, become accustomed to the pain, the passive motions suitable to the joint may be begun.

E'

"The adhesions existing within and around the joint may be of so firm and resistant a nature as to readily lead to the belief in the existence of bony ankylosis. At first the amount of motion obtained in the joint will be exceedingly small, but even with this we will be bound to rest satisfied, for an increase of mobility often does not begin for months; in the meanwhile the patience of both physician and patient will necessarily be put to a severe test. Nevertheless, keeping in mind the old saying, that 'constant dropping wears away the rock,' treatment must be continued steadily and systematically.

"The astonishing results which experienced mechano-thercopists often obtain in cases declared incurable by others can often be explained by the consistent and methodical treatment which they pursue.

"The knee-joint is very often the seat of extensive synovial exudation in consequence of chronic rheumatism. Resorption is to be effected as in synovitis in general, namely, by centripetal stroking, pressing, and kneading."

The following is an interesting case of stiffness of the right shoulder which the writer treated a few years ago:—

A rather feeble lady, about forty-five years of age, was struck on her right forearm. There was no fracture nor sprain, but the arm was kept in a sling for two months. Then the lady found that she could hardly move her arm at the shoulder-joint. The adhesions were broken up. During the operation the shoulder was mechanically dislocated and reset. Inflammatory adhesions followed, and the operation was repeated with no better result. The joint was stiff, with great inflammation of the deltoid and the adjacent nerves and tendons, and so tender and sore that it could not be touched when the physician prescribed massage.

The patient being under the influence of an injection of morphine administered by the physician, the writer was enabled to apply treatment consisting of centripetal kneading and stroking. After a few days the injection was discontinued and passive motions were applied, in addition to the manipulations. Two weeks later active and resistive movements were used. After two months' treatment the patient was well.

SPRAINS.

In this class of diseases this mode of treatment has scored one of its greatest successes.

In treating a sprain of the ankle we begin with gentle *centripetal stroking*, commencing at the toes and gradually proceeding upward to the knee. If the pain does not allow of touching the diseased part, it will be best to begin the stroking from above the painful point and gradually begin from a lower point till at last we shall be able to apply the stroking all over the ankle. As the pain diminishes more and more force may be employed, and *kneading*, *circular*, and *vibratory friction* be applied.

This manipulation should be continued from seven to fifteen minutes twice a day.

After the third or fourth sitting the movement of the ankle-joint will generally be quite free and almost painless, and *passive flexion* and *extension* and *rotation* should be performed, soon followed with *active* and *resistive flexion* and *extension*.

Provided there is no fracture, four to ten days is enough to cure the patient when the treatment is begun at once. If it has been allowed to go on for months and even years, this treatment will still prove to be most effective, and in the average of these old cases a cure may be effected in from one to three months.

Other joints are treated on the same plan.

The hip- and shoulder- joints are more difficult to treat and require a much longer time in order to produce a cure.

The following cited cases are especially noteworthy:—

CASE I. A gentleman, thirty-six years old, sprained his right ankle by a fall, and had been on crutches for eight months, when he came for treatment, May, 1883. There was no flexibility of the ankle, which was very tender and swollen. After six weeks' treatment once a day the patient was cured.

CASE II. A young lady had come to Washington to see the inauguration of President Cleveland in 1885. Three weeks before, she slipped on the icy pavement and sprained her right ankle. She was laid up, and all sorts of liniments, etc., were prescribed by her physician. After ten days he told her that there was nothing more to do but to keep quiet for two or three months, when she probably would be well. At this point the writer was called in, and the young lady told him, with tears in her eyes, why she had come to the city, and that now she was told that she would have to be quiet in her room for

months, and she implored the writer to do his
best. The ankle was still black and blue and
very much swollen, and the pain did not allow
of touching the parts. After the examination
she was informed that she would probably be
well in ten days if treatment was applied twice a
day. To this she was only too glad to con-
sent.

The treatment was given twice that day. The
next day the most of the discoloration had disappeared, and now she was told to walk a little
at a time in her room. The improvement was
remarkable from day to day. The ninth day
after, the seventeenth sitting, she was cured, and
went to the inauguration ball on the tenth day.

She had no relapse.

CASE III. About two years ago one of the
writer's assistants sprained his left ankle in a
gymnasium. He was brought home by his .
friends and told to be quiet in bed. He kept on
all night bathing the leg with hot and cold water,
and came next morning to the Institute. The
joint was slightly dislocated, the foot was turned
upward and inward, and twice as large as usual.
The patient was a strong young man, so that the
writer at once went to work and succeeded in

getting the joint straight, after which a full treatment was applied.

After four days' treatment, twice a day, the young man was well.

Prof. Dr. J. Nicolaysen, of Christiania (in *Norsk Mag. for Lægevidenskab*, 1874), communicates the following case of *hydrarthrus* (water on the knee) :—

" A man, thirty-two years old, had suffered from hydrarthrus for six and one-half years. Repeated punctures and evacuation had always been followed by a re-accumulation of the fluid.

" Massage was used for several months, and the patient returned to his work. There was no relapse."

Another gentleman, twenty-six years old, had suffered from hydrarthrus for two months, when he came to the same professor, who sent him to the writer, at that time in Norway.

After two weeks' treatment the collection of fluid in the knee-joint disappeared, but the swelling of the capsule continued.

After five weeks' treatment the patient was well.

INDEX.

9 781436 738583